THE 168 HOUR CAREGIVING WORK WEEK:

ACTIVITY AND BEHAVIOR INTERVENTIONS FOR LOW FUNCTIONING INDIVIDUALS

Activity Ideas For:

- ☉ Alzheimer's Disease
- ☉ Lewy Body Dementia
- ☉ Parkinson's Disease
- ☉ Stroke
- ☉ Frontal Lobe Dementia
- ☉ Huntington's Disease
- ☉ Traumatic Brain Injury
- ☉ and more

Silknitter, Keegan, and Duretz

Disclaimer

This book is for informational purposes only and is not intended as medical advice, diagnosis, or treatment. Always seek advice from a qualified physician about medical concerns, and do not disregard medical advice because of something you may read within this book. This book does not replace the needs for diagnostic evaluation, ongoing physician care, and professional assessment of treatments. Every effort has been made to make this book as complete and helpful as possible. It is important, however, for this book to be used as a resource and idea-generating guide and not as an ultimate source for plan of care.

ISBN 978-1-943285-28-0

Published by
Caregiving 101

Quick Guide to Activities and Behavior Management for the Low Functioning

The 24/7 job of caregiving for a low functioning loved one can be challenging. No matter the cause — dementia, traumatic brain injury, stroke or something else — finding and adapting the ideas to engage your loved one in an activity or learning to work with a behavioral outburst is hard.

This book is designed as a quick guide for ideas to get you started.

Throw away any pre-conceived notions you and others may have on how something should be done. There is no right or wrong way when it comes to activities. There is only what works for you and your loved one.

Table of Contents

Activities for the Lower Functioning

No matter the reason — a form of dementia, a brain injury or something that happened at birth — if your loved one's cognitive and physical function are low, engaging them in some form of leisure or daily living activity will be beneficial. The keys to success are knowing your loved one's:

- Past and personal history
- Strengths and weaknesses
- Interests and preferences

Knowing these things will allow you to choose and plan activities that meet your loved one where he or she is and better allow for successful completion of a chosen activity.

Before we look at activity ideas to help, let's review three important areas that you must be mindful of to give yourself the greatest opportunity to engage your lower functioning loved one. These three areas are: Flexibility, Planning and Benefits.

Flexibility

Please know that your ability to be flexible and go with the flow is an important part of the process when working with someone who has Alzheimer's or any other form of dementia or is lower functioning.

Here is an example of what we mean. Billy loved to play Euchre. As his Alzheimer's progressed, he forgot the rules and would often make up new rules to the game. The family had two choices. They could spend their time correcting Billy each time he did something wrong, or they could go with the flow and just enjoy playing and watching the look on Billy's face when he won every game.

Planning

Whether the activity involves playing a game or bathing, pre-planning as many details as possible can make a significant, positive difference for everyone. Interactions that may start with one activity can lead to others. For example, looking at a photo album may prompt a discussion about a family reunion, which could lead to a discussion about a wedding, and then a discussion about a song that was played at your loved one's wedding. Little things matter. You never know where an activity or a conversation can take you.

Knowing a person's strengths and weaknesses will also assist in meaningful activity and behavioral changes. Concentrate on the activities your loved one can do and the most appropriate times for her to do such activities. If your loved one is more energetic in the morning, then physical activities would be most beneficial then. If she is more agitated in the afternoon, that's when the less strenuous, more relaxing types of activities, such as listening to or playing favorite music, or being read to might be more appropriate.

Know your own strengths and weaknesses as well. When do you need a break? What do you enjoy doing?

Know the strengths and weaknesses of individuals who will help with your loved one. If you know that the friend coming later in the day has a special interest in reading the Bible, then leave that for the friend to do with your loved one.

Benefits

<u>Caregiver Benefits</u>

Planned and well-executed activities can result in less stress for you and your loved one. It may also give you that little bit of time to yourself while the person you care for is engaged in an activity.

When your loved one is actively engaged and participating in a reminiscing-type activity, such as looking at pictures in photo albums, chances are your loved one will relax. This in return gives you, the caregiver, the same opportunity to feel relaxed. It also provides an opportunity to converse and reminisce about past experiences.

Social Benefits

Engaging loved ones in a variety of activities can have the same positive effects that they experienced through positive social interactions throughout their entire lives.

Intellectual Benefits

Any type of activity that allows an individual to think and come up with a response
allows for a more meaningful interaction and is
then beneficial to both the caregiver and the loved one.

Emotional Benefits

It just makes us "feel good" to have a pleasant interaction with another human being. Think about your life and all of the evenings out
with friends you have had over the years, when you were having so much fun that you did not want the night to end. Just because someone has Alzheimer's does not mean

that his reaction to positive interaction will be any different.

Spiritual Benefits

Socialization during spiritual activities can help to ensure that one's belief system remains fluid throughout the transitions of living. Bible studies, prayer groups, prayers, and other services that support the need to connect and those that provide fellowship can be very beneficial. These activities help maintain and even strengthen faith and hope and may even provide an understanding of existence.

Physical Benefits

The old adage of "use it or lose it" comes into play with regard to the physical functioning of individuals. The more your loved one exercises and does physical types of activities, the better it is for her overall health and well-being. No matter how simple an activity may seem to you and others, make sure to encourage your loved one to do it.

Self-Esteem Benefits

Leisure activities which are offered at the right skill level provide your loved one with an opportunity for success. Any time we can do something for ourselves, we feel better than having someone else do that task for us. Small or large, from brushing teeth to creating original art pieces, each of us enjoys the satisfaction and resulting praise from accomplishing something.

Sleep Benefits

Alzheimer's disease and sundowning can play havoc with an individual's sleep patterns. Engagement and activities can have a direct benefit to sleep patterns for everyone. The more active a person is during the day, the more likely the person may be to sleep better throughout the night.

Behavioral Benefits of Activities

Well-planned and well-executed activities of any type can reduce challenging behaviors that sometimes arise when caring for someone with dementia.

Behaviors are nothing more than a means of communication when words are no longer effective. Keeping this in mind allows you, the caregiver, to find understanding when a behavior occurs and to potentially recognize triggers for certain behaviors.

This knowledge is particularly important as working with behaviors is one of the most challenging issues caregivers face.

Prepare multiple activity interventions and have the resources you will need to execute them ready and close by as you never know exactly when your loved one might encounter something that triggers a behavior.

While reading through and using any of the activity suggestions offered here, please remember that nothing works forever. As your loved one's issues progress and abilities decrease, you must take note of what has changed and make modifications to allow your loved one to continue to enjoy an activity. You must also make sure to keep everyone who meets your loved one updated on any changes that you have perceived in your loved one.

Music Activities

Music can engage your loved one, by stimulating memories or changing a mood. Below are tips and multiple activities for you to try that involve music.

Use a person-centered approach and music that interests your loved one. There are many genres to choose from and your loved one may like several of the following:

- Blues
- Classical
- Country
- Dance
- Easy Listening
- Electronic
- European
- Gospel
- Punk
- Hip-Hop
- Holiday
- Inspirational
- Jazz
- Latin
- New Age

- Opera
- Patriotic
- Pop
- R&B/Soul
- Reggae
- Rock
- World Music

Music Tips

Before getting started with playing music, please remember:

- Follow TAPAS. Play music in the right TIME AND PLACE AND SITUATION.

- Tell your loved one what is happening, so as to not startle the person when the music begins.

- Your loved one may not be able to tell you exactly how he feels about the music so watch for reactions.

  - If you see happiness, you can confirm it by asking questions about the song.

- If you see sadness set in, you should ask if there is anything about the song that is upsetting and whether it is better to stop the music.

- Be sensitive to when you ask the person for confirmation as to whether the music is pleasing. If he becomes agitated if you speak during a favorite song, wait until the song is over to ask.

Music Delivery Methods

There are several options to deliver music to your loved one depending on what you have available to you and what you can afford to purchase. Options include:
- Old records played on a turntable
- Cassettes played on a tape recorder
- A radio
- A computer
- Music videos watched on websites, such as YouTube or Vimeo
- MP3 Players
- Tablets
- Smartphones, such as Apple iPhones or Samsung Galaxy

Smartphones, Tablets, MP3 Players and Computers

These devices provide the best opportunities to provide music for our loved ones. We can create playlists of favorite songs, artists and styles of music. We can offer music anywhere at any time.

A playlist is simply a list of songs or performances that play one after the other without interruption. When creating a playlist for your loved one, here are some tips:

- Shorter playlists can be better than longer ones, so you don't overdo it.

- Create multiple playlists for different times of day, activities and moods. Examples include:
    - Calming playlist
    - Energetic/upbeat playlist
    - Cooking playlist
    - Morning playlist — To help us wake up
    - Afternoon playlist – For fun

- Evening playlist – To slow us down
- Holiday playlist
- Favorite artist playlist
- Gospel playlist
- Visitor playlist – To play when another caregiver or family is visiting
- Sing-A-Long playlist

The possibilities are endless. Please take the time to create the playlists, so they are ready to go at a moment's notice.

Headphones, Earbuds or Speakers

When using smartphones, tablets, MP3 players or computers, there are multiple ways to deliver the music to your loved one which you must choose from depending on the situation and what is needed at the specific time.

- Speakers are a perfect way to fill a room or a home with music. Wireless speakers using Bluetooth technology allow you to carry a small speaker from room to room.

- Do not use earbuds.

- Use over-the-ear headphones and remove hearing aids.

  o Adjust volume to a comfortable level for your loved one.

  o If your loved one cannot speak to communicate, read her body language and facial expressions to tell you if the music should be turned down.

  o Do not leave your loved one unsupervised as she may not be able to turn off the music or think to remove the headphones when wanting to stop listening. This could lead to a negative behavior.

Please remember to use "listening to music" as just one of the several activity tools you use to engage your loved one. Music, like anything, can become less effective if it is overused.

Singing Music

Singing or humming a song is an excellent activity to engage your loved one. Here are some tips:

- Create playlists of songs that your loved one is familiar with.

- Join him in sing-a-long songs, and try being the first to sing to provide an example if your loved one is not singing.

- Watch movie musicals together and sing along.

- Sing hymns and gospel songs.

- Have a kitchen band with pots and pans or utensils.

Music Games and Activities

- Play finish the music lyric games.

- Play Name That Tune by humming or singing songs your loved one knows.

- Look up favorite musicians and songs on the internet.

- Reminisce about the music of childhood.

- Exercise to music.

- Learn and try different dance styles to popular music genres. Many of these can be adapted to be done in a chair.

- Write a new verse to a favorite song.

- Use blank music sheets to create a new piece together.

- Discuss music from your loved one's entire life: what music was popular when she was 20? 30? 40?

- Discuss favorite artists from the age she thinks she is, e.g., if she believes she is 25 years old, use popular singers or songs of that era.

- Discuss music chosen for and played at weddings.

Baby Doll Nurture Program

This program works when everyone that meets your loved one is on the same page. A Baby Doll Program is more than just handing a low functioning individual a Baby Doll. A Baby Doll Program can give an individual purpose and a reason to get up and moving in the morning. It can be the thing that gives that person an incentive to wake up in morning, take care of her personal needs, and have her breakfast.

Let's look at Mom. Mom was a quiet lady, with dementia, who stayed in her pajamas and lay in bed all day, even when family and friends came to visit. Mom would sit up to eat meals brought to the bedroom and always had the television on. The only real stimulation she had or was interested in were visits to her room from family and friends or when the kids brought their dog over.

As we mentioned at the beginning of this book, one of the keys to successfully engaging your loved one is knowing her past and personal history. If Mom loved being a mom and loved to nurture both young and old, then a Baby Doll program might work for her.

To get started, you can look at multiple ways to introduce the Baby Doll to Mom. One way is to bring a Baby Doll into the room and place it off to the side, in plain sight, while encouraging Mom to get dressed. You can choose to start on a day when you have visitors coming or must leave the house for an outing, so she can be given a reason to get dressed. Help her as needed. If, while dressing, she looks at the Baby Doll and asks who it is, tell her that it is a baby visiting for the day. After Mom is dressed, help her sit and place the Baby Doll on her lap. Ask her if she would mind holding the baby or taking it for a stroll.

Mom may ask what the baby's name is, or she may immediately start calling the Baby Doll one of her kid's names, such as Joseph. Just go with it as Mom may believe the Baby Doll is a real child or one of her kids.

Like many who have benefited from a Baby Doll Nurture Program, Mom may begin to change a little each day. She may stop lying in bed all day. With regular encouragement and assistance, Mom may get up, get dressed, and go out of her room with Baby Doll Joseph.

As with any program, there may be unplanned consequences that you must watch out for. For example, if Mom starts leaving her room and eating meals in the dining room, she might bring Joseph, her baby son. She might sit him on her lap, talk to him, and not eat. She may scream if you try to take Joseph away. To help, explain that Baby Joseph needs to go to the nursery to be changed and fed. You can then encourage Mom to eat while Baby Joseph is being taken care of. Explain to her that you will bring him back as soon as everyone is fed and cleaned up.

Another issue which may arise is that Mom may not want to go to bed. She may want to be with Baby Joseph 24/7. To help, you can use the same strategy of going to the nursery. Explain that Joseph needs to go to the nursery to sleep as all babies need their sleep to grow. You can also comment on how exhausted she must be as it is your understanding that most mothers of young babies get exhausted from providing constant care. Encourage her to get some rest, and assure her that if Joseph needs anything through the night, you will take care of him.

Please remember that the key to success is that everyone must be on the same page for the Baby Doll Nurture Program. This includes Dad or anyone else who might think it is inappropriate for Mom to carry a doll. They need to put those pre-conceived notions away, and allow mom to enjoy the baby. If they can, they will see the benefits of Mom's being engaged and happy as well.

General Activities for Low Functioning Adults

A library of activities to choose from is essential for any caregiver. If you use any of the activity suggestions below, please make sure you have all the materials available and ready to go for each activity. Be prepared to modify the activity to your loved one's abilities.

<u>Activity Boxes</u>

To make it easy for you or any caregiver working with your loved one, you can build and label Activity Boxes. Activity Boxes are individual containers that have the necessary items for a single activity. By assembling multiple Activity Boxes, all caregivers will be prepared to engage their loved ones at a scheduled time, or in times of crises or behavioral outbursts, to redirect loved ones' focus in order to re-establish a sense of calm.

Items for activity boxes may include the following:

- Dominos or games, such as Connect 4

- Playing cards, memory/matching cards or conversation cards
- Adult or children's coloring books/templates with crayons, markers or colored pencils
- Topic specific trivia, questions or discussion points
- Large piece jigsaw puzzles
- Locks and keys, large nuts and bolts or PVC pipe pieces, sandpaper and wooden blocks
- Pick-Up sticks
- Small musical instruments
- Scarves to touch and try on
- Knitting and crochet items
- Items to make a tie blanket
- Tools and materials for manicures
- Tools and materials for hand massage
- Tools and materials for pedicures
- Tools and materials to shine shoes
- Tools and materials for flower arranging. (For example: Use a spaghetti strainer and fake flowers. Let

your loved one arrange the flowers through the holes.)

- Tools and materials for clipping coupons to have a magazine scavenger hunt
- Play-doh or kinetic sand
- Sensory bottles, I spy bottles, Discovery bottles
- Materials to stuff envelopes
- Old photos and scrapbooks
- Items for sorting
  - Large buttons
  - Poker chips
  - Decks of cards – First sort black and red cards and then by suit if the person can. Then sort face cards from numbered cards.
  - Plastic cutlery
  - Ribbons, laces or wool
  - Different fruits to be put in specific bowls
  - Different sets of colored balls to be put in matching color trays
  - Socks

- Napkins – Fold once they are sorted
- Hand towels – Fold once they are sorted
- Color match using colored folders and colored paper. Have them put the colored paper in the matching colored folder.
- Greeting cards
- Vintage jewelry
- Coins
- Colored clothespins
- Craft pompoms
- Pasta shapes
- Cereal pieces
- Items for stacking
  - Paper or plastic cups
  - 3-D bingo chips
  - Sponges
  - Buttons
  - Jenga game pieces
  - River rocks
  - Tupperware

Reading Activities

For these activities, the intent is for you or another caregiver to read to your loved one. Try reading different genres from the following list:

- Magazine articles on topics of interest to your loved one
- Happy books
- Children's books
- Western books
- "Dear Abby" articles from newspaper
- Horoscopes
- Joke books
- Magazines and catalogs for scavenger hunts
- Inspirational stories
- Animal stories
- Chicken Soup for the Soul books
- Erma Bombeck, Jerry Apps, Phyllis Diller, Beatrix Potter books

Writing and Coloring Activities

- Writing
  - Address envelopes
  - Write name
  - Place hands on a clock to tell time

- Coloring
  - Use crayons or pencils
  - Use coloring books or print templates from internet
  - Photocopy personal pictures for a feeling of familiarity

Writing and Coloring Activity Tips

- If your loved one has trouble holding a pen or pencil, wrap foam around the shaft of the pen to help your loved one's grip. You can try cutting a piece from a foam noodle used in a swimming pool to fit on the writing tool.

- Reduce glare and shadowing by positioning a chair and table so any natural light is behind them instead of coming at them from the front.

- To prevent shadows, place lamps on the opposite side of the hand being used.

- Locate the bottom edge of the lampshade just below eye level.

- Shiny paper can increase glare, so it's
best to use matte paper when reading or writing.

Note: Know the type of seating where your loved one is the most comfortable when he is writing, and, if possible, move him to that seat.

Note: If your loved one is seated in wheelchair, recliner, or bed, provide a flat surface that fits in his lap to place paper on.

Pet and Animal Therapy

Several studies have shown the benefits gained through pet-assisted therapy in long-term care facilities. Those same benefits can be enjoyed with a pet in the home. They include:

- Experiencing companionship and unconditional love

- Providing a purpose when your loved one cares for the animal

- Improved socialization and interaction opportunities

- Improved eating habits

- Reduced anxiety

As caregivers, we must match the best type of pet with the abilities of our loved one. If we are caring for our loved one at home, we must also have someone as a backup to assist with caring for the pet should things become difficult for us or for our loved one.

Spiritual Activities

Spiritual activities can mean different things to different people. Make sure you know what works with your loved one.

<u>Religion</u>

There are many religions. For this book, we will use examples from Christianity.

- Praying
- Reading the Bible
- Praying the Rosary
- Reciting the Lord's Prayer
- Discussing religious symbols and their meaning
- Holding and touching religious symbols
- Singing Hymns
- Finishing the Bible Verse — say the beginning part of a well-known Bible verse, and let the participant finish the rest
- Finishing the Hymn — say a part of a famous hymn and allow your loved one to finish the line.
- Listening to Bible stories

- Listening to Mass or a religious service on the television or radio
- Listening to church bells, organ music, and piano music
- Reminiscing about significant religious and spiritual experiences from the person's life

Natural and Artistic

- Sitting outdoors
- Listening to positive visualizations or guided mediations
- Spending time in the garden
- Bird-watching
- Stargazing
- Poetry
- Inspirational stories
- One-on-one visits with pastors, rabbi, clergy, etc.
- Nature sounds
- Viewing artwork
- Creating artwork
- Sensory gardens

- Aromatherapy

- Deep breathing

- Nature videos

Crystals

Some believe that crystals can provide multiple benefits and can be worn, carried, or placed in your home. In addition, you can use the crystals as a sensory activity where your loved one can hold different textured pieces in her hands. The following are a couple of suggestions of what some people believe are the helpful properties of particular crystals:

- To balance mind, body and spirit while reducing hostility and agitation:

  o Agate

  o Bloodstone

  o Carnelian

  o Chert

  o Flint

  o Jasper

  o Onyx

- ○ Sardonyx

- To remove negative energy in all the chakras; reinstate loving, gentle forces of self-love; bring calmness and clarity to emotions and restore mind to harmony after chaotic or crisis situations:
  - ○ Rose Quartz

- To assist with aging in general; encourages clarity of mind:
  - ○ Blue Kyanite
  - ○ Rutilated Quartz

- To ease fear and depression and create balance between body and emotion:
  - ○ Botswana Agate
  - ○ Lepidolite

Reminiscing Activities

A staple of any program to engage low functioning adults are reminiscing activities. When trying one of the following, do not ask "Do you remember?" Just explain what you will be doing, bring the materials out, and begin. Here are some ideas to help:

- Reminiscing boxes – Fill a box with topic-specific items from a time or moment in your loved one's life or from an activity which she enjoyed doing. This can include:
  - Military service
  - Past occupations
  - Cooking
  - Jewelry box
  - School days
  - Childhood
  - Tools
  - Woodworking
  - Sports once played
  - Weddings
  - Favorite vacations

- Photo albums and family photos

- Create a puzzle. Use magazine or printed pictures of kids or pets, cut them into 4 pieces or 5 pieces (or more depending on the person's skill level).

- Junk Drawer – Ask the person to help you find items that you've lost in the drawer. Many of us had "Junk Drawers" in our homes to put things that had no other place to go but could not be thrown away. Gather items, create a list, and ask for his help in locating items. Use a bin or a box if you don't have an extra drawer lying around to use. Reminiscing opportunities include:

  - What was in your loved one's junk drawer?

  - Where was the junk drawer located in his home?

  - How often did it get cleaned?

- Cooking. If Mom cannot perform many of the tasks to make a meal, ask her to help you with one of her favorite recipes. Let her direct you and see what types of conversations arise. Does she talk about that meal or people who once enjoyed eating it?

Reminiscing Discussions

Reminiscing discussions are a fabulous and inexpensive way to engage. The following topics are great starting points:

Colors

- Colors of favorite sports team

- Colors chosen for wedding

- Colors of flowers or cars

Military Service

- War stories — if this is a topic your loved one is comfortable discussing and he wants to recount events

- World events of his time

- Personal experiences of either military service or what it was like in the United States during another era

Holidays

- Specific holidays that coincide with your loved one's culture or religion

- Favorite holidays and holiday traditions

- Most memorable holiday memory

Cooking

- Home cooking

- Comfort food

- Favorite recipes from Mom/Grandma

- Favorite food associated with events, holidays, family gatherings

- Making a cookbook with loved one to pass on to the family

Sports

- Favorite professional sports teams

- Previous involvement in sports

- Big sporting events from former eras

School Days

- Where your loved one went to school

- Favorite subjects, classes or teachers

- Activities and clubs she was in

- Memories of her children's school events

Old Cars

- The family's first car

- Your loved one's first car

- Prices of cars now and then

- Dream cars

Travel

- Places traveled

- Favorite vacations

- Monuments and special places visited

Family

- How your loved one met his spouse

- Father's occupation; mother's occupation

- Favorite meals

- Vacation spots

Pets

- Pet names

- Pet characteristics

- Funny pet stories

- Life on a farm

Dancing

- Learning to dance

- Barn dances, Dance Halls, & Dance clubs

- Romance on the dance floor

- Popular dance songs

- Popular dance styles

Friendship

- Childhood friends

- Lifelong friends

- Best qualities in a friend

- Pen pals

- Activities done with friends

Hobbies

- Favorite things to do for fun

- Memberships in clubs or organizations

- Activities and sports while at school

- Hobbies shared with a spouse

Recreational and Outdoor Activities

- Ball or balloon toss

- Watch children create chalk drawings

- Blow bubbles

- Wiggle toes in the garden dirt, sand box, or kiddie pool

- Take the dog outside or visit the neighbor's dog

- Plant a sensory garden

- Plant a container garden

- Plant seeds

- Create bird feeders with toilet paper tubes, peanut butter, and birdseed

- Enjoy eating a meal outdoors

- BBQ

- Picnic

- Meditate in a garden

- Fill the bird feeder

- String popcorn or cereal for the birds

- Sit in the sun (wear sunscreen!)

- Relax in the shade

- Use a metal detector

- Watch the neighbor kids play in the yard

- Fly a kite

- Feed the ducks

- Play yard games

- Visit an apple orchard

- Harvest the garden

- Deadhead the flowers in the garden

- Watch the birdhouse or birdbath

- Name that bird call

- Watch the clouds

- Have morning coffee or afternoon tea outdoors

- Make sun prints with photo paper

Computer Games and Activities

Advances in technology have opened worlds of possibilities to engage our loved ones. Whether you are using a computer, tablet or smartphone to access the internet, there are an increasing number of options for you to use. Here are some examples:

Computer Games

There are many games which you and your loved one can enjoy on computers, tablets or smartphones. With the advancement of touch screen technology, your loved one can enjoy interactive games simply touching the screen. Examples of online games include:

- Tic Tac Toe

- Match images

- Dress up

- Paint and Color

- Use a pottery wheel

- Name that Tune

- Card Games

- Digital versions of board games

- Checkers

- Color match games

- Identify the object

Computer Activities

The number of activities you can do using the internet and technology are only limited by your imagination and access. Some great activities to consider are:

- Armchair travel – Research locations and places of interest and discuss interesting facts

- Play Where in the World — Use Google Street View to search and find:

  o Your loved one's first home address
  o Where she went to school
  o Where she was married
  o Places she has traveled
  o Places she would like to travel

- Research recipes to cook with

- Research information on favorite sports stars

- Research information on past hobbies

- Listen to free music on allmusic.com

- AKC.org for dog lovers

- Listen to live air traffic control at www.liveatc.net

- View fine art at www.artcyclopedia.com

- View "Today in History" at www.infoplease.com/yearbyyear

- Watch upcoming movie trailers at http://trailers.apple.com/trailers

- Reminisce while listening to television show introductions at www.tv-intros.com

Art Activities

- Wrap bubble wrap around a paper towel tube, roll onto an ink pad, and stamp on paper for great designs.

- Cut various fabrics into squares and/or rectangles, and arrange them onto a sheet of paper to create a fabric quilt.

- Wrap yarn around a small block of wood, dip in paint, and use as a stamp.

Sensory Activities: Smell

Smells are a great way to engage your loved one and help him through his day.

Aromatherapy is based on the principle that natural fragrances, or essential oils, from certain plants or flowers can affect our moods.

Essential Oils and Moods

- Stress Relief
    - Bergamot, Chamomile, Lavender, Lemon, Orange, Patchouli, Vanilla, Ylang Ylang
- Anxiety/Fear
    - Bergamot, Chamomile (Roman), Cedarwood, Frankincense, Jasmine, Lavender, Neroli, Patchouli, Rose, Sandalwood
- Self-Esteem
    - Bergamot, Cypress, Grapefruit, Jasmine, Orange, Rosemary
- Sadness/Grief
    - Bergamot, Chamomile (Roman), Clary Sage, Frankincense, Grapefruit, Jasmine, Lavender,

Lemon, Orange, Rose, Sandalwood,
Ylang Ylang

- Fatigue
  - Basil, Bergamot, Clary Sage,
    Frankincense, Ginger, Grapefruit,
    Jasmine, Lemon, Patchouli,
    Peppermint, Rosemary,
    Sandalwood

- Agitation
  - Chamomile (Roman), Lavender,
    Mandarin, Sandalwood

Essential Oil Applications

- As an activity. Place drops of essential
  oils on cotton balls, and put cotton
  balls in small plastic containers. Pass
  containers around to identify scents.

- As an activity, small scented sachets
  can be used as well. Place a small piece
  of pillow/craft stuffing on a small fabric
  square. Scent the stuffing with a few
  drops of preferred essential oils. Tie
  the sachet with pretty ribbon.

- As an activity, mix preferred essential
  oil with unscented lotion. Place
  rubbing lotions on wash cloths and

pass them around. Talk about what the smells remind you of.

- As an activity, create smelling bottles by placing a couple of drops of baking extracts or essential oils onto cotton balls, and then place into small, individual bottles.

- As an activity, squish wax with lavender in your hands; pass the wax to your loved one. It's great for arthritis and helps relax and hydrate the hands.

- For a calming moment, burn a candle scented with the desired essential oil.

- For calming moment, place a scented candle into a glass jar and then place the jar on an electric cup warmer.

Note: If your loved one is allergic to any essential oil, do not use it.

Note: Do not apply drops directly to your skin; blend with carrier oils or lotions if you want to apply it that way.

Fruit

- Cut open fruit and let your loved one hold, smell and maybe eat the fruit.

- Savor oranges and lemons by rolling them, cutting them in half, and then squeezing the juice out. Enjoy the aroma.

- Puree different fruits in a food processor to create edible paint.

Spice and Baking Scents
- Place spices like cinnamon, nutmeg, and oregano on a cotton ball. Place the cotton ball in a small plastic container and pass it around allowing everyone to enjoy the aroma.

- During fall and winter, keep cinnamon sticks, orange slices, cloves, and maybe some apples in a pot with water on the stove. Heat as needed to activate the aroma.

- Bake cookies.

- Bake treats like lemon cake, gingerbread men, strawberry cake, pies, and Bundt cakes.

- Bake seasonal recipes. For example, in October, you can enjoy the smells of the season by making pumpkin muffins, Crock-Pot veggie soup, or Crock-Pot apple cider.

- Brew coffee or herbal teas.

Garden Scents

- Place different herbs in small covered boxes. Each person picks a box to guess which herb is in the box and discusses what the smell reminds her of.

- Flowers. The same activity for herbs can be used for different flowers.

- Make fruit infused water by filling a pitcher to the top with ice and fruit. Fill the pitcher with cool water. Let sit for at least one hour. Poking holes in the fruit helps to release the flavors faster. Some tasty and unique smelling flavors include:

kiwi-orange, raspberry mint, strawberry basil, cucumber lemon, and blueberry lime.

- Create delicious herbal drinks by infusing lemonade with herbs from the garden. Try lavender, rosemary, elderflower, or watermelon-basil. Smell first, then sip.

- Do you have mint in your garden? Freeze whole mint leaves into ice cubes. You can also mince the herbs and pack them into an ice cube tray, until about ¾ full. Fill the tray with hot water and carefully place in the freezer.

- Create herb butter by pouring either extra-virgin olive oil or melted, unsalted butter over herbs. Cover the container lightly with plastic wrap and let freeze overnight.

Sensory Activities: Touch

Sensory stimulation uses everyday objects to arouse one or more of the five senses: hearing, sight, smell, taste and touch. The goal is to evoke positive feelings.

Here are some ideas for sensory activities using touch:

- Holding and squeezing foam pieces

- Holding different textured fabrics and materials like silk, cotton or velour

- Hand massages with scented lotions

- Manicures and pedicures

- Foot baths

- Warm or cold compresses

- Brushing hair

- Shoulder rub

- Scalp massage

- Find the Special: Hide sweets, treats or items in a large bowl of cooked spaghetti. Ask individual to be brave and put their hand in to find the "Special" item.

- Shuck corn

- Peel cucumbers or carrots

- Mash potatoes

- Wash dishes

- Snap peas

- Tear lettuce

- Cut fruit

- Cut hard-boiled eggs

- Mix baking ingredients

- Create 'Moon Sand' by mixing eight cups of flour and one cup of baby oil. The mixture is extremely soft and easy to mold into shapes.

- Wind yarn around a hoop and string beads onto the end of the yarn to create a dream catcher.

- Create sensory bags with sealable plastic bag filled with hair gel and

small, soft items which will not puncture
the bag.

- Make scented soap

- Make fake snow

- Fill a bowl with different dry ingredients, such as dried beans or large grains. Have your loved one, separate the different items and place in different bowls.

Sensory Activities: Sight

Sight can be as simple as your loved one looking at colorful swatches of fabric, pictures or colored paper. When using images, avoid patterns that are too busy or pictures that are too complex.

Internet Videos

- Animal videos
  - o Puppies
  - o Kittens

- Live webcams from zoos and aquariums

- Laughing baby videos

- "How To" videos from home repair to cooking

- Music and dancing videos

Please note that with tablets and smartphones you can find videos on the internet to watch and then project them on to your television with products like Apple TV.

Sensory Activities: Hearing

Sound therapy can be used to help reduce stress and change a mood. Often, natural sounds, such as running water or birdsong work well.

Using music, as described in the earlier section of this book, is a great tool.

Note: Individuals who have difficulty processing sounds can find relatively quiet noises distracting and aggravating.

Behavior Examples and Interventions

Medication has its place and can be a valuable tool when working with behaviors. We must always consult our loved one's medical team when behaviors are happening which we do not understand.

Remember, behaviors are nothing more than a means of communication when words are no longer effective.

For example, the pain and discomfort of a UTI may cause your loved one to constantly get up from a chair and try to leave the house to get to the doctor on his own. He may not be able to tell you what is happening and what he is trying to do, so you may think he is just trying to wander off.

In another example, our loved one's dementia may have robbed the memories of the last
50 years so that she thinks she is a young 23-year-old wife and mother. She may be constantly calling out and looking for her

little baby girl, because when she was 23 you were a one-year old child. We should try to understand the trigger of a behavior, so we are not tempted to use medication to keep someone quiet or calm for our convenience.

Interventions to Utilize to Mitigate Aggressive Behaviors

Activities can help when challenging behavior occurs. They can be used as a form of redirection, such as going for a walk, moving into another room in the house, or focusing on what is on the walls, like pictures.

Distraction can be most helpful. Never disagree, argue, or ask your loved one to remember something. Caregivers can often control difficult situations by distracting their loved one. They can also work to avoid events or triggers of bad behaviors.

For example, if a person gets agitated by the sound of the garbage truck collecting trash once a week because it is a faint, but disruptive noise, the caregiver can make trash day a day for a favorite activity, such as listening to music. Trash pickup day could then become a "good day" for your loved one.

Skeletons in the Closet

Please note that there is no special intervention that works immediately. It may take hours or days or weeks or months to find interventions that work regularly and for more than a few minutes.

Many families do not know about a trauma that their loved one experienced in her youth. These traumas can turn into behaviors that we do not understand. Once families find out what happened to Mom, it may help adult children understand why Mom behaves a certain way or why she did certain things or set certain rules while they were young.

A great example is that of an 82-year-old woman who one day became terrified of showers. She would scream blood curdling screams when anyone tried to help her shower or bathe. This was an ongoing battle while the family and her doctors tried to figure out what was causing the screaming.

Eventually an outside caregiver hired by the family to help Mom and give the grown daughter a break began building a relationship with Mom. The caregiver knew Mom used to play the piano and was able to get her to sit at the piano to play a song while the caregiver sang. While this was happening, the caregiver would touch her hand and try to be friendly. Mom only had the one daughter, so the caregiver called her "mother of one" which always made her smile.

The caregiver would escort Mom around the house as needed, but would let Mom "assist" her instead of the other way around — giving Mom a purpose and the feeling that she was caring for the caregiver.

As the trust and relationship grew, the caregiver suggested that Mom get cleaned up, as it had been a few days since she bathed.

The caregiver helped Mom into the bathroom, started running the water to get it warm, and put towels on the floor and shower seat to remove any potential chill Mom might experience when she stepped in and sat down. She then gave Mom the shower hose and allowed her to control the water. This meant a lot of cleaning up afterwards, but Mom was in control.

After months of this routine, Mom turned to the caregiver one day after the shower and said, "She didn't drown today." The caregiver said, "You saved yourself," and Mom said, "Yes." They sat for a moment and Mom began to tell the story of "the boy who put his thing there and then tried to drown me."

The caregiver later explained what she had learned to Mom's daughter, who had no idea that happened to her mother. That explanation also helped the daughter understand why Mom would not go to any lakes or swimming pools herself or allow the daughter to go either when she was younger.

Daily Log

One of the best tools a caregiver can use to identify a trigger for a behavior is a daily log of your loved one's day. In addition to watching for health changes, such as a UTI or reactions to a medication change, your log should include things, such as:

- Who he came in contact with.
  - Did family or friends visit?
  - Did a caregiver or personal aide who Dad built a relationship with not show up as scheduled?
  - Did a speech therapist who you know he doesn't like come to work with Dad?

- Change to her daily routine.
  - Did she miss the morning news?
  - Was she able to have her evening cup of tea before bed?
  - Did she have her after-meal smoke?

- Exposure to violence
  - Was there a violent program on TV?
  - Is there a major weather event happening somewhere in the world being discussed on the news?
  - Did he see visitors, such as grandkids arguing?

- Change in environment
  - Did new neighbors move in with a dog that barks constantly when left outside?
  - Is there an unfamiliar noise outside, such as contractors putting a new roof on the neighbor's house or road work being done?
  - Is there an unexpected glare from the morning sun because blinds were adjusted by someone in the house?

o Is there a change in temperature causing her to be too hot or too cold?

Behavior Examples

Here are examples of behaviors that many caregivers have experienced and some ideas to help.

Aggressive Behavior: Screaming

Example 1: Screaming for attention or help

Your loved one begins screaming out for Mommy or Daddy or asking to be helped continually whether in her bed or dining room or family room.

Example 2: Screaming, "I can't get out of here!"

Your loved one starts moving from room to room and door to door trying to get outside to go somewhere while screaming.

Many seniors experienced extreme trauma in their youth, and with dementia, they may be re-living the experiences.

Someone may have been raped and told to keep quiet so as not to disgrace the family. Others may have been beaten up in their youth. Some may have been lost in a store, and others may have been locked in a closet. The point is, your loved one may believe that traumatic events which happened over 50 years ago may be happening again.

First, we need to make sure the person is safe and that he is not being or has not recently been sexually assaulted, beaten or locked in his closet. Once we have confirmed that he is not in danger, we can validate his feelings and offer comfort while figuring out what is triggering the behavior.

We need to know why she is calling for her parents or why he is trying to get out.

We must understand that dementia allows us to peek into early life events of our loved one which we never knew about.

Center yourself, stay calm, and if it helps, approach the situation as if the person who is suffering is yourself. This allows you to meet your loved one where she is for a better understanding of what she is physically and emotionally experiencing at that moment.

For best results, know as much of your loved one's personal history as possible — his wants, his needs and his preferences. Let everyone who helps with caregiving duties know as well. With dementia, nothing stays secret and in the closet forever. Get things out in the open to help all caregivers as well as your loved one.

General Intervention Best Practices

- First observe for pain, discomfort or a medical issue.

- Once pain and discomfort or a medical issue is ruled out, identify the trigger.

- While working to identify the trigger, validate the person's feelings and let her know you understand.

- Stay calm and do not argue with her.

- Address any physical needs, such as toileting, hunger or thirst.

o Redirect your loved one by asking her to help you get something to drink while you work on her issue together.

Intervention Activity Tips for Screaming

- Pet therapy or pet interaction with live animals. You can also use interactive animal dolls that purr or move as someone pets them.

- Play music from a calming playlist you have created.

- A warm shawl and a stuffed bear to cuddle.

- A walk outside or to another room in the house

- Offer sensory items and activities with soothing smells.

- If your loved one is nurturing by nature, offer a baby doll for her to watch over and help.

Time and Place Orientation: "I Want To Go Home"

Example 1: A father with dementia had been living at his son's house for two years. Recently, Dad started standing by the door, with his bags packed, yelling, "I want to go home!" or "This isn't my house." or "When are we leaving?"

Wanting to go home is common for someone with Alzheimer's or dementia who can no longer safely live on his own and has moved in with family or to a nursing home.

<u>General Intervention Best Practices</u>

- First observe for pain, discomfort or medical issue.

- Once pain and discomfort or a medical issue are ruled out, identify the trigger.

- While working to identify the trigger, validate his feelings and let him know you understand.

- Stay calm and do not argue with him.

- Address any physical needs, such as toileting, hunger or thirst.

- Validate and redirect your loved one by asking him to help you pick out a snack before the trip.

- Validate and redirect your loved one by saying that if you are going anywhere, you need to use the restroom first. Suggest that your loved one use it as well before the trip.

Intervention Activity Tips for Time and Place Orientation

- Offer valid reasons why you can't leave at that moment, such as:

  - We can't leave until later because … the traffic is terrible.

  - We can't leave until tomorrow because … the forecast is calling for bad weather.

  - We can't leave until tomorrow because … it's too late to leave tonight.

- Use the "home" she wishes to go to as a topic for reminiscing by starting with the statement, "Ok, but what does the house look like?"

- Discuss the features of the house, and let those features lead to other reminiscing discussion points.

  o What color is it? What color would you like it to be? What is your favorite color?

  o Is there anyone home? Who lives there with you? Tell me about them. What was your Mom/Dad like?

  o Is it close to any building, like a church or a school? Where did you go to school? What was your favorite part of playing football in high school?

  o Does it have a garage? What was your first car? What is your favorite car?

Aggressive Behavior: Hitting or Biting and Swearing

Aggressive behaviors can be defined as hitting, angry outbursts, biting and angry swearing outbursts. It can be scary for a caregiver to provide care to someone who is aggressive. Just like any other behavior, aggressive behavior is nothing more than a means to communicate what the client can no longer say with words.

An example to consider is the father with dementia who had been living with his son for two years. One day Dad stood by the door yelling, "I want to go home! This isn't my house. When are we leaving?"

Wanting to go home or saying "I do not live here" is common for someone with dementia who can no longer safely live on his own and has moved in with family or to a nursing home.

General Intervention Best Practices

- First observe for pain, discomfort or medical issue.

- Once pain and discomfort or a medical issue is ruled out, identify the trigger.

- While working to identify the trigger, validate her feelings and let her know you understand.

- Stay calm and do not argue with her.

- Address any physical needs, such as toileting, hunger or thirst.

  o Redirect your loved one by asking her to help you get something to drink while you work on her issue together.

Possible Causes for Aggression

- Too much noise/overstimulation

- Cluttered environment

- Uncomfortable temperatures

- Basic needs unmet (toileting, hunger, thirst)

- Pain

- Fear/anxiety

- Confusion

- Communication barriers

- Scared because he does not recognize his surroundings

- Caregiver's mood

- He perceives that he is being rushed

Interventions to Use with Aggressive Behaviors

- Engage and redirect through an activity, such as:

  - Play music from a calming playlist you have created.

  - Introduce calming sensory smells, such as lavender by asking the person to help "identify the smell" or just placing a diffusor with calming essential oils in the room.

  - Use spiritual support and activities if important to your loved one.

- Reminisce using specific details of her past and topics of interest to her, such as cars, kids, colors, flowers, weddings.

- Offer items of comfort, such as a picture of the family.

- Provide consistent caregivers and caregiver schedules. Stick to the client's routine.

- Plan recreational activities that match her abilities and interests as tolerated.

- Break down instructions to one-step increments.

- Help the client slow down and relax.

- Play music from a calming playlist you have created.

Repetitive Speech or Behaviors

Example: Repetitive behaviors can manifest as repetitive movements, sounds and words. Typical repetitive behaviors can be repetitive questions, words or phrases; clapping or rubbing of the hands; pacing, often accompanied by a dusting or wiping motion; or rummaging through drawers and closets.

One caregiver shared the story of her father and how Dad repeats everything, talks to himself, making statements like, "I gotta go. I gotta go!" or "I can't go! I can't go!" Sometimes he counts out loud.

When they are at home, the family and caretakers just let him walk up and down the hallway, and eventually he calms down. But when not at home, they sometimes struggle with Dad's repetitive behaviors. Sometimes they can just tell him it's okay, and he'll calm down and ask if they are sure. Other times, that does not work.

There is always a reason for such behaviors; there is always a story behind them. When discovering the hidden story or source, you will have a chance at resolving the behaviors.

Sometimes it is a simple thing you don't think of that can help. Other times, you may go through a series of intervention steps before finding one what will calm him down.

Following are some intervention engagement tips that can distract, redirect, and help calm the person while you are working to find and remove the trigger. For best results, know as much of your loved one's personal history as possible — what she might need or want and what her preferences might be.

- First you want to observe for pain or discomfort. Once pain and discomfort are ruled out, the other possible cause could be overstimulation. Create a quiet, calm environment by removing environmental barriers that could be contributing to the overstimulation.

- Once it's determined that the behavior is not causing harm and your loved one is not in pain, accept it and stay calm.

- Address both physical and social needs starting with toileting needs if needed.

- Offer magazines with pictures based on topics of interest.

- Start a discussion by asking open-minded questions to promote conversation by:

  o Using topics the person can relate to and reminisce about.

  o Talking about his strengths and skills.

  o Giving him sincere praise.

- Provide a drink, such as lemonade and a snack while talking with him.

- If during your discussion, he starts asking the same question over and over, answer each repeated question as if it is the first time.

- Be aware of your body language and tone when answering questions.

- Offer tactile or comfort items to enhance sensory stimulation. This can include:
  - A weighted or stuffed animal
  - A soft blanket
  - Items he can roll in his hands
- Offer activities that are repetitive in motion, such as coloring or sorting and folding clothes.
- Offer sensory touch activities, such as:
  - Hand massages
  - Scalp massages
- Focus your loved one's attention on emotionally soothing activities, such as:
  - Listening to music
  - Singing lullabies or hymns
- Entertainment activities, such as:
  - YouTube videos
  - Internet games and activities

o Watching favorite movies and TV shows, like *The Sound of Music* or game shows

Inappropriate Sexual Expressions

Sexuality in the elderly often receives little attention or education. Being aware that inappropriate behavior can manifest itself in a sexual nature will prepare caregivers to identify and react properly to a loved one exhibiting these behaviors.

Example 1: An adult daughter is the primary caregiver for Dad. Dad thinks that his daughter, who is the spitting image of her mother, is his wife. Mom has been Dad's primary caregiver for years but became ill herself and passed. Dad went to go live with his daughter as he could not live by himself. The daughter quickly realized that there were times that Dad thought she was Mom by comments that Dad made or how he tried to touch her.

You may also see the following behaviors manifest in a person suffering from dementia:

- Behaviors expressed publicly without regard for others

- Touching others sexually without being able to discern if the desire is mutual

- Inability to verbalize 'Yes' or 'No' to sexual advances

- Misinterpreting touches, smiles, and hugs as sexual invitations

- Engaging in sexual acts with someone who is not her spouse or companion

- Disrobing or urinating in inappropriate places

- Sexual comments or gestures that might be offensive to others

- Fondling or masturbating in inappropriate places

- Unreasonable jealousy or suspicion

Interventions for Inappropriate Behaviors During Personal Care

- Step back from your loved one, creating a spatial barrier.

- Use a calm, firm tone of voice.

- Call your loved one by his surname to get his attention, creating a formal boundary.

- Identify yourself and your function/intent.

- Beware of your body language.

- You may need to excuse yourself from the room. First make sure your loved one is safe and explain that you will return in a few moments to resume care.

Intervention for Inappropriate Behaviors in Public Areas

- Remove your loved one from the public area.

- Provide privacy in an appropriate area.

- Provide comfort items as necessary.

- Maintain dignity — no teasing or shaming.

General Interventions

- Check for a possible urinary tract infection

- Check for genital skin irritations

- Check for uncomfortable clothing:

  o Too tight or small

  o Too loose

  o Too bulky if the client is wearing multiple layers of clothing

- Model and encourage nonsexual forms of intimacy

- Use a fanny pack or tool belt filled with items to distract someone who is fondling clothing below the waste or around genital areas.

Poor Judgment: Hoarding

Hoarding is the consistent behavior of accumulating and storing objects that the person perceives are necessary to keep.

Example: The person collects food that is rotten not realizing that consuming such food could be harmful to himself and others he might offer the food to.

Concerns Associated with Hoarding

- Falls due to clutter

- Fires in the home-care setting

- Medications misplaced due to clutter or hiding the items

- Respiratory ailments due to dust and mold and dirt

- Rodent or insect infestation

- Ingestion of rotten food or something toxic or harmful

Possible Causes for Hoarding

- Items perceived to be valuable

- Items provide a source of security

- Fear of forgetting or losing items

- Fear of being robbed

- Anxiety disorder

- Obsessive compulsive disorder

- Depression

- Constant need to collect and keep things

- Obtaining love not sensed from people

Interventions

- Decide if the hoarding is harmful/unsafe and remove unsafe items, such as rotten food.

- Use a soft, gentle approach.

- For early stages psychological support might be an option.

- Go slowly and expect gradual changes.

- Don't force interventions. If you need to clean out the room or a drawer where hoarding is evident, wait until the person has left the area.

- Don't be critical or judgmental.

- Don't press for information that is making your loved one uncomfortable.

- Don't make negative, teasing, or sarcastic comments.

Hallucinations and Paranoia

Paranoia is an unrealistic belief accompanied by feelings of persecution, blame and suspicion.

Example 1: Mom sees spiders on the walls of her bedroom at night and begins screaming and banging on the wall.

Example 2: Dad sees and hears kids running around the house and keeps yelling at them to be quiet. Some days, he tries to chase them through the house and falls.

If this is a new behavior for your loved one, and you have ruled out any medical illness as a contributing factor, then look at sensory-related issues.

- If your loved one wears glasses, make sure they are clean and not broken.

- If your loved one wears hearing aids, make sure they are functioning properly with fresh batteries.

- Pay attention to environmental contributors, such as:

  o Loud or soft noises

o   Is there proper lighting with no shadows?

Approaches and Interventions to use

- Reassure your loved one that she is safe and you are there to help.

- Use gentle touching when appropriate to turn her focus to you and away from the hallucination.

- Speak in a calm, soft tone, and find out the details of the situation.

- Assure your loved one the situation will be corrected.

- Move to a different, well-lit room if needed to calm her down.

- Once she is calm, conduct further investigation to re-establish a stable setting.

- Repeat activities proven to be successful, such as:

    o   Music activities — use the calming playlist you created

- Use calming sensory activities, such as calming essential oils in a diffuser or holding her hand to let her know she is safe.

- Involve her in familiar, work-related activities.

- Involve her in physical activities to burn energy.

- Provide activities that are repetitive in nature.

Resources

With over 300 activity ideas to get you started, this book is just one tool available to caregivers who struggle to get their loved ones to stay active and live the highest quality of life possible.

There are thousands of websites, books, support groups and companies to support family caregivers around the world.

There is no right or wrong answer when it comes to engaging your loved one. The key is to make the effort and be ready to adapt all activities to your loved one's abilities.

We know that caregiving is a struggle. Be strong and never give up.

*9 7 8 1 9 4 3 2 8 5 2 8 0 *